HIV/AIDS AWARENESS

HIV/AIDS IS NOT A DEATH SENTENCE

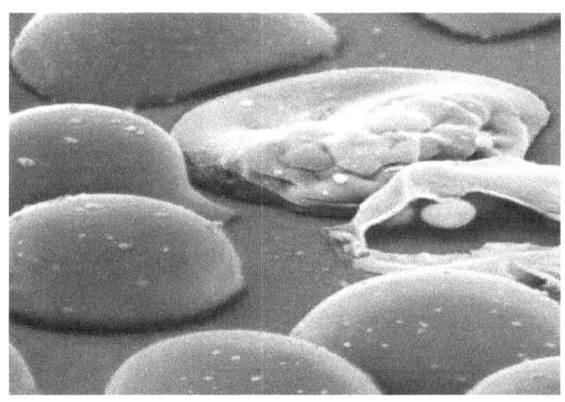

By Beverly Hill

Introduction

I want to thank you and congratulate you for choosing the book, *"HIV/AIDS AWARENESS: HIV/AIDS IS NOT A DEATH SENTENCE"*.

When the Human Immunodeficiency Virus (HIV); was clinically noticed in 1981, in the United States. The news of such a dreaded virus took people around the world like a thunder storm.

The fear of the fact that there was no cure, and no one knew the capacity of which the virus could assume a dual nature of a living and non-living thing, and the reality that the virus could be passed on was very worrisome then. The initial case study was about impairment noticed in some gay men with no known reasons why they had a strange syndrome of pneumonia which was very rare at that time.

What is HIV? The Human Immunodeficiency Virus is a long virus belonging to a member of the subgroup of retrovirus, which is the virus that causes HIV infection, and also causes the acquisition of the corresponding immunodeficiency syndrome (AIDS). AIDS is a conditioning in human beings in which gradual failure of the immune system permits life threatening infections to thrive. If there is no treatment given to an infected person, an average survival period after infection with HIV is estimated to be between 9 to 11 years which also depends on the category or subtype of the HIV group the person is infected with.

There are many misconceptions of the subject matter of HIV/AIDS. But the fact is that this book will put the record straight, and tell you the real truth about HIV/AIDS. So you need to understand that the virus cannot be transferred, and you can live a long and happy life if you follow the simple steps listed in this book.

Thanks again for choosing this book, I hope you enjoy it!

ABOUT THE AUTHOR

Beverly Hill is a sociologist. She is the CEO of C.E.F Associates and formerly served as head of department of sociology in Premier Natural Resources Inc.

A graduate of Nelson High School also graduated from the University of Toronto with a B.A in economics and finance and holds an M.S from Cambridge University in public relations and PhD in sociology.

She has written many articles on human equality, animal rights, environmental issues, personal development and peace keeping in different newspapers. She has also appeared in many magazines and is frequently interviewed for articles on family, race, socioeconomic status, and how to survive in your environment. She has also worked on the importance of health of relationship between parents and children. Her book 'The Middle Child' focuses on the importance of the attention given to the children and what to expect from them. This book helps parents understand their children.

In addition to these works she is also the author of 'Surviving Alone ' which is about her own childhood growing up; she writes about her family struggles living on a low income budget and growing her own food to survive.

C.E.F Associates formed in 1999 in Idaho, USA she worked both nationally and internationally. This is a consulting company which has clients all over the world. Ms. Hill the CEO of the company is the main reason of the huge client base because of her servings in foreign countries.

TABLE OF CONTENT

Conclusion

Preview Of 'MIDDLE AGE CAREER CHANGE: How To Turn Your Life Passion Into A Career'

Chapter 1: MIDDLE AGE CAREER CHANGE

Chapter 1

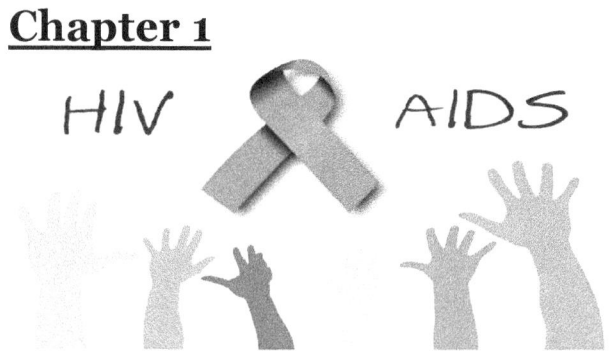

THE FULL MEANING AND OPERATION OF HIV/AIDS

When we are talking about Human Immunodeficiency Virus (HIV) as described above, there is a particular condition that the virus will constitute in the human system, and that is, it will continue to attack the body cells of the infected person, and the body will be defeated, or wear down and this subjects the body to another condition which is even more critical, and worst than the virus itself, and that is AIDS. AIDS means Acquired Immunodeficiency Syndrome (AIDS), the syndrome is a gradual and successful failure of the human immune system which further allows, and give the opportunity to other infections to thrive, and easily destroy the immune system and bring it to a devastating, dilapidated and finally kills the infected person.

Diseases that easily thrive with a person who has Acquired Immunodeficiency Syndrome (AIDS)

Cancer

An HIV/AIDS infected person whose immune system has been weakened by the final stage of the infected virus will tend to actually lose the fight when the AIDS condition of the person has gotten to a critical level, and this can be referred to as the "breaking point" when the body system cannot resist or fight back to stay alive. There are other diseases that can also easily have their way when a person is infected with AIDS diseases such as pneumonia, tuberculoses, yellow fever, and swine fever.

Chapter 2

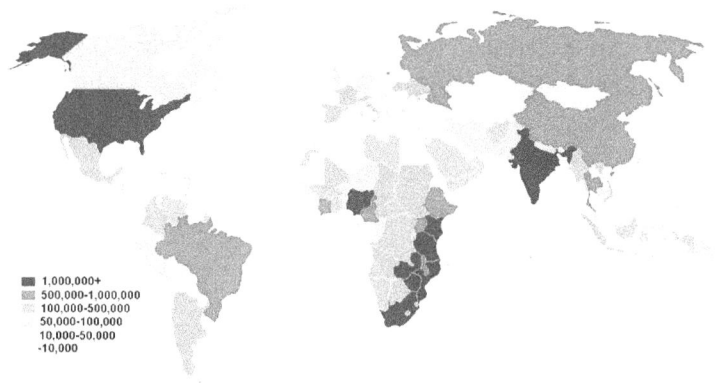

IMPORTANT FACTS ABOUT HIV AND AIDS

The HIV virus attacks the T-cells in the human immune system, while AIDS is only a syndrome which appears or emerges in the advanced stages of the HIV infection.

HIV is a virus infection, while AIDS is a medical condition.

In the vast majority of cases the HIV always leads to the AIDS condition if it is not treated at the early stage with anti-retroviral drugs etc.

No known cure for HIV/AIDS

It can take a toll on those who are infected with HIV/AIDS finding life very difficult.

Average cost of treating a person with HIV/AIDS is estimated to be in the region of $379,668 throughout the person's lifetime. How many can sustain this? Your guess is as good as mine.

The worst case of HIV/AIDS is between Africans and Americans than any other race.

New and common infections are prevalent among nursing mothers, women and children via unsterilized needles etc.

Chapter 3

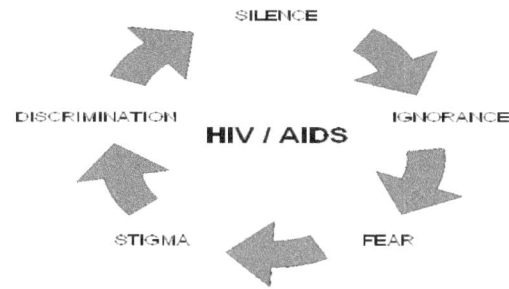

THE ORGIN OF HIV

It was the belief as put forward by scientist that both the HIV1 and HIV2 type originated from non human primates in West and Central Africa, and somehow through interactions, or contact made, it was transferred to human brings through a process called zoonosis in the earlier part of the twentieth century. The HIV1 type was first discovered in the bodies of Chimpanzees from the Southern Part of Cameroon. The HIV2 type was discovered living in the body of an old monkey that lived in littoral Western Africa particularly the Southern part of Senegal through the West coast of Ivory Coast. It was also discovered that the Owl Monkey was resistant to the HIV1 type virus as a result of their inherent genomic fusion of two different viral restraint genes.

The Erroneous believe about HIV

The many misconceptions on the subject matter of HIV are very many. But the fact is that this book will put the record straight, and tell you the real truth about HIV. So you need to understand that the virus cannot be transferred or transmitted through any of the following means viz-a-viz.

Shaking Hands with infected person

The virus cannot be transferred to any person if you just had a handshake with an infected person contrary to the erroneous believe of some people who think that HIV can be transferred via a hand shake.

Hugging an Infected Person

If you hug someone that is HIV positive you cannot contact the disease, since the virus has to do with the immune system of the person mere hugging such a person does not take you into the person's immune system, you are no fluid. So you don't have to be scared HIV is not a death sentence.

Casual Kissing an Infected person

There is no way you can contact HIV by kissing someone who has an infection or pecking an infected person contrary to the erroneous believe that the virus can be contracted by doing so.

Touching unbroken Skin of an infected person

Using the same toilet with a HIV positive person does not make you a victim of a death sentence, so there is no need to think you have been infected when you use the toilet that is already used by an infected person.

Although every person needs to maintain personal hygiene, sharing towels with an infected person however, does not transmit the virus to such a person.

Either mouth to mouth resuscitation

May be you are trying to revive someone who has fainted, this does not transmit the virus if you do so, or any other form of casual contact does not cause you to contract HIV. So go ahead and live your normal life without fear of death, just keep the above principle and tips in mind.

Chapter 4

HIV CAN BE TRANSMITTED THROUGH...

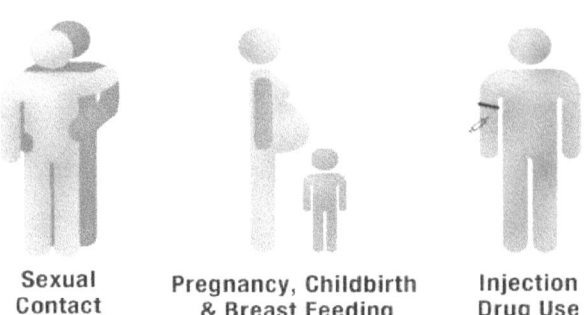

Sexual
Contact

Pregnancy, Childbirth
& Breast Feeding

Injection
Drug Use

MODE OF TRANSMISSION OF HIV

Semen: HIV is a sexually transmittable disease, in fact the most common and foremost means of contracting HIV is through sexual intercourse or unprotected sex. Once an infected male or female, lets says a male for instance (who is infected), engages in sexual intercourse with a female, the male's released sperm cells carries along with it the virus, and once he introduces it into the body of the female, the female will contact the virus. As a result of sexually transmitted diseases the procurement of condoms was being produced and released to further checkmate the spread of deadly diseases. However, scientist and many professionals in the health and private sector of the contemporary societies have continued to argue about the potency, or ability of condoms to protect a person from contacting HIV. There are many submissions that condoms cannot guarantee maximum protection from HIV, and the experts canvassed for total abstinence as the best means of avoiding infection.

Blood: This is a very critical mode and means of contacting the HIV disease, once the virus finds its way into the blood stream of any human being that is very dangerous. Because, at the time the virus was noticed and discovered, apparently there was no visible cure for the virus, and the means of protection against such virus was not readily available and ascertained until later on as time passed, scientist were able to discover drugs that could reduce some of the destructive capacities of the HIV.

One of the means that an individual can contact this dreaded diseases is **via blood transfusion.** In hospitals for instance, there are patients who go for medical treatment of one ailment or the other. And if the patient is not well taken care of because of negligence on the part of the medical personnel in charge of the ward for giving the requisite for treatment. Accident victims or patients who are undergoing surgery may require blood to be donated, and transfused into their body system as a result of shortage of blood in their body, and if the blood donor is not properly screened to see if his system is void of HIV, until proper screening is done, no blood transfusion should be-allowed to be administered on the patient. So one of the means of contacting the HIV disease is through blood transfusion, that is, if the blood is infected with HIV.

Virginal fluid-pre-ejaculation: It is also observed that HIV can also be transmitted from female to a male via virginal fluid prior to ejaculation by the male via sexual intercourse; hence, both parties are liable to contact the disease. Persons who are sexually promiscuous without the idea, or self control in terms of morals are susceptible to be infected. There are ongoing awareness campaigns from both government and nongovernmental organizations all over the world that regularly canvass the dangers of engaging in illicit sexual activities that will tend to spread, and cause HIV infection.

Breast Milk: A mother who is infected with HIV is capable of transferring the virus to her baby through breast milk. Millions of children are dying every day as a result of HIV infection from nursing mothers. This situation has been putting more pressure on the little facilities available in the hospitals, and the government is having a hard time containing the malicious, and chronic HIV disease which is plaguing some people around the world today.

Sharing of Sharp objects such Razor Blades or needles: A blood stain sharp object like razor blade, needles, clippers etc. can lead to HIV infection, when the blood stains are made to come in contact from an infected person to a person who is not infected. Any contact made will cause a transmission to be effective. That is the reason it is always recommended that needles and clippers be sterilized before usage.

How the HIV operates in the body system: HIV syndrome is a serious body cell attacking infection which consistently attacks the immune system of the body, which is the stronghold of the virus. When this happens, the individual's immune system will be weakened, and any minor or major ailment will succeed in attacking the individual whose immune system has been shattered by HIV.

Common ailment like malaria, tuberculoses, yellow fever, and any other type of sickness will further have the power to succeed when it feast on an infected person. So the HIV virus attacks and paves the way for further devastative effect of other diseases.

Chapter 5

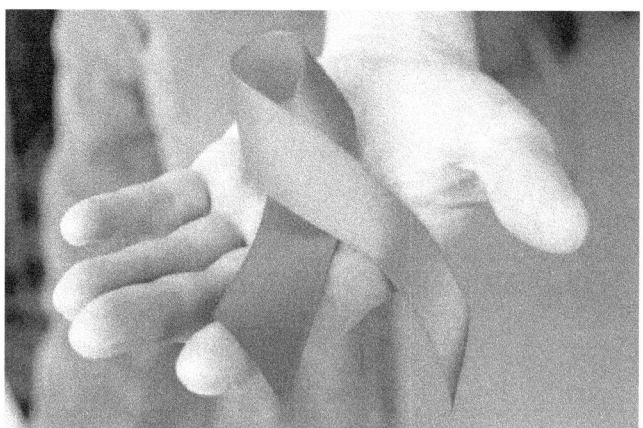

WHY HIV IS NOT A DEATH SENTENCE

Contrary to the initial believe that HIV is a killer disease, I mean, people still have the fear and superstition that HIV is an instant killer. Today we have seen that this belief was very wrong because of the result, and the fact that there was said to be no found cure for the dreaded diseases up till now, there is no confirmed cure for HIV. Scientist is still working hard to develop a drug that will finally put an end to the deadly virus.

Improvements have been made in the field and continuous research for the cure for HIV. There are drugs that have been developed that halt, or mitigate the activities of the virus causing HIV/AIDS commonly referred to as the retroviral drug. These drugs work by reducing the dangerous activities and attacks of the virus. There are individuals who have been able to manage the virus in their system for as long as twenty years, and yet have not died from the HIV infection.

A famous basket ball player in the United States who was infected with HIV over twenty years ago is still alive. He was able to manage his situation with the assistance of medication (i.e. the anti-retroviral drugs). Hence, it has been successfully demonstrated that the fact that a person his HIV disease is not mean a death sentence. While some people who get the knowledge that they have been infected are devastated and become demoralized. Infected persons who always feel this way further harm themselves by developing psychological trauma, suffer depression etc. which further negatively affect their health.

Infected persons can still have relationship with the understanding that they can continue to live their lives without hitches, or any form of fear of the unknown or death. It is important that infected persons adhere to medical advice, and feel free to live their lives or enjoy their lives without having to have the apprehension of a sudden death. It has been proven on several occasions that embracing someone who is infected with HIV do not transmit the disease. The major means of infecting a person has already been discussed above, but the major ways of causing infection is through unprotected sexual intercourse, sharing of sharp blood stained objects with an infected person etc.

Why many people think being "HIV positive means death sentence", is the fear of death itself. Also, the overhyped and over-exaggeration of the HIV disease from inception went a long way to further poison the minds of the people against the plague. For instance, in third world countries especially in Africa, the alleged infection has continued to increase in millions from the Eastern, Western and Southern Africa the figure of infected persons presented is in millions, it is not that other parts of the world are exempted, Asia Europe, America etc. also have people with HIV/AIDS in large numbers too, but the ability to control it; continuous research and discoveries of new ways to halt and contain the activities of the virus, such that people are able to go on with their various business or way of life without fear of any sudden death as long as they keep to their medication they are able to live a healthy lifestyle this is why it has made the difference between the third world countries and developed countries.

The third world countries also have some of the facilities that can assist in containing the virus, but the fact remains that due to continuous increase in the number of infected person, and coupled with the fact that the population of infected persons continue to add pressure to the limited facilities on ground is not helping matters.

There are people who are HIV positive, and are afloat enough to afford the vaccines, or retroviral drugs that can help them to stay alive and healthy without a sign of weakness or infection, they are still happy, and are living a normal life style. So being HIV positive is not a death sentence, it is only an awareness that you need to take more care, and be concerned about your health, and take good care of yourself and above all live a happy life.

Chapter 6

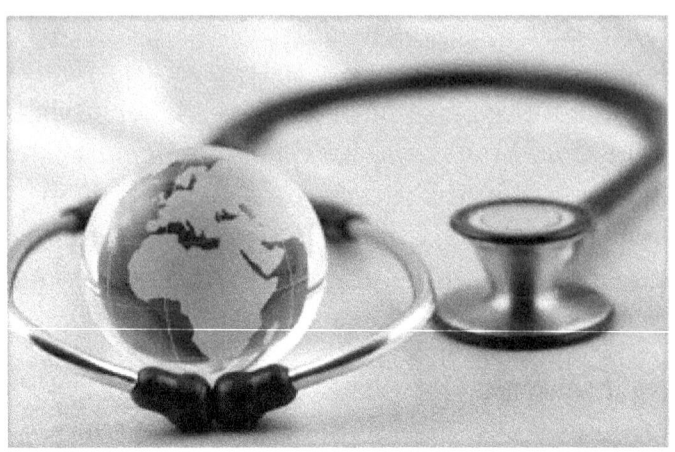

WORLD HEALTH ORGANIZATION (WHO) POSITION ON HIV

The World Health Organization in its documents on the subject matter of HIV/AIDS has stipulated that government at all levels, and also private individuals are being encourage to work towards the halting of the spread of HIV, and also work towards creating awareness of the existence of the deadly virus, and carry out awareness campaigns to sensitize its people about HIV. It has stressed that it is not good that infected persons are being ostracized in some countries. It further stressed as a matter of fact, that those who are victims should be cared for, and shown much love.

The World Health Organization also stated that the fact remains, that if a person is infected, there need not be any fear of immediate death, but that available means of taking care of the health situation should be deployed, or administered to the infected person such as the retroviral drugs which will help to retard the activities of the virus, and thereby enabling the individual who is infected to be able to live longer.

It has also urge governments of various nations to work towards the acquisition of the retroviral drugs at a subsidized rate to be made available to infected persons in the hospitals, and that will be a step in the right direction in bringing a measure of control to the spread, and further bringing to the minimal level of the population infected with the virus.

Hence, with these activities of the World Health Organization (WHO), and with the efforts of all stake holders involved in providing health care, it is crystal clear that there should be no need for anyone to panic, and understand the fact that when a person is infected with HIV, it does not mean death sentence to such an individual.

Chapter 7

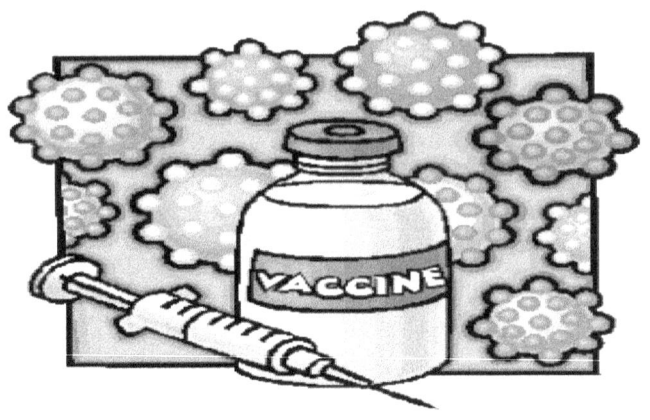

GOVERNMENT EFFORTS AT ASSISTING HIV INFECTED PERSONS

In line with the World Health Organization's policies on the urge for effective implementation of HIV screening and health care centers, government at all levels have continued to intensify efforts over the years to see that it complies with the modalities presented by World Health Organization on treatment of HIV infected persons.

General Hospital belonging to the government has departments who are taking care of infected persons, and also the necessary vaccines like the retroviral drugs, and the likes are being dispensed at a subsidized rate which can be readily available and accessible by HIV infected persons.

There's efforts being made by both the international organization like WHO, nongovernmental organization, and also the government at different levels is significant reason why someone who has the virus should not think that having it is a "DEATH SENTENCE," No! not at all! Some persons who have been infected have continued with their lives, and have been living for years simply because they were able to manage their situation very well.

Chapter 8

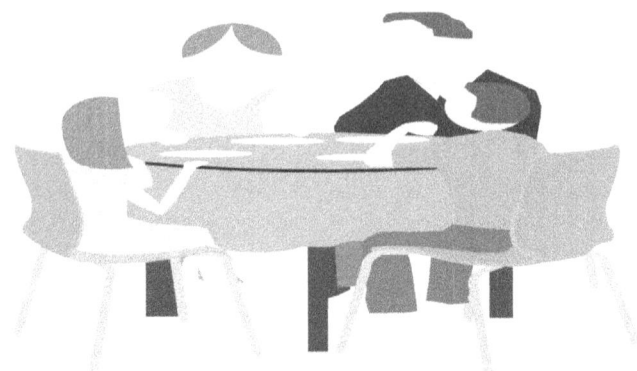

HIV INFECTED PERSON CAN STILL LIVE A NORMAL LIFE

Contrary to the adverse believe that HIV infected person are doom to death, is a blatant lie, it has been proven and established that infected individuals can always live as long as they can live if they can take good medical care of themselves by taking the medical advice, and checkup on regular basis.

HIV infection should not warrant any fear of death whatsoever. It may be quite a surprise and saddening experience that you are made to face the fact that you are HIV positive, but then, life goes on, you don't need to embark on retaliation, because that is what some people do. They go about spreading the virus through unprotected sex with a vengeful intent. There is no justification for embarking on such mission.

But rather, look at your actions in another perspective, like we have seen infected persons who have come out to openly admit to the fact that they have been infected, and they go on to establish Non Governmental Organization to assist others who have been infected with the HIV diseases or even partnering with the government, or World Health Organization to campaign an created awareness about the scourge of HIV. Now! That is a positive way to start, and it will even maker the infected person a lot more happier and fulfilled without the regret that he or she has been infected; when the person looks back and see how many lives he or she has been able to touch and inspired by helping others to overcome the erroneous beliefs that they are doomed to death.

Conclusion

Thank you again for choosing this book!

I hope this book was able to help you to understand HIV/AIDS is not a death sentence.

It is true that the scourge of HIV is real, but the simple truth is that HIV does not mean a death sentence to say the least. Any person who is HIV positive can still go about living a normal life, and awareness should be created by all stake holders to continue to sensitize the people who have the erroneous belief and myth that HIV is an instant death sentence which is not true.

The only observation that should be noted is that the medical condition that HIV leads to which is AIDS is a more advanced stage of a situation that has gotten out of hand. Aids is when the immune system of a person has been weakened, and gives ways for further attacks by other diseases, or other dangerous medical condition like cancer etc. which finally kills the sick person.

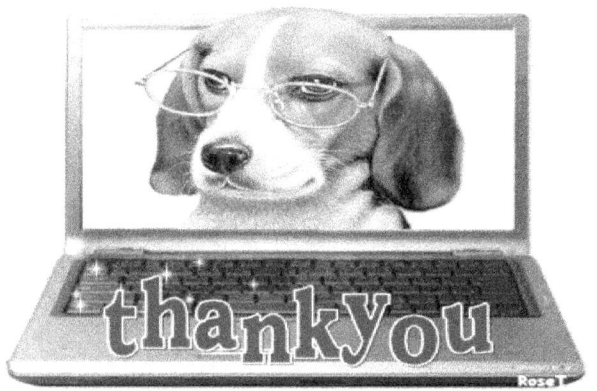

Finally, if you enjoyed this book, would you be kind enough to leave a review for this book on Amazon? It'd be greatly appreciated!

Thank you and good luck!

Preview Of 'MIDDLE AGE CAREER CHANGE: How To Turn Your Life Passion Into A Career'

Chapter 1: MIDDLE AGE CAREER CHANGE

In a economy limping along with a high percent unemployment rate, it's not unusual for even the gainfully employed to test free agency and see what else might be available. In a 2009 Salary.com survey, when global financial markets were still plummeting, more than 65 percent of workers said they were actively looking for new jobs.

It's one thing to change jobs, something most people will do more than 10 times between the ages of 18 and 42, but it's quite another to change careers. Making the leap from a field in which you've been trained and have experience to a wholly new one takes careful consideration planning and the right expectations.

This is true of anyone interested in making a change, but what about professionals who have been in the workforce for 20 or 30-plus years? Baby boomers, born between 1946 and 1064, make up 40 percent of the labor force, and shifting gears later in life to focus on new career objectives can be challenging, but also rewarding. Seasoned professionals often have a different perspective than their younger colleagues.

Middle-aged workers usually place more value on nonmonetary benefits, such as less stress, flexible work schedules and personal fulfillment, so when they're able to change careers they can make the jump to areas that are more professionally fulfilling rather than having to worry about how much they earn.

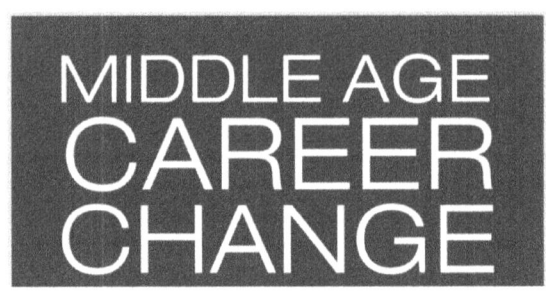

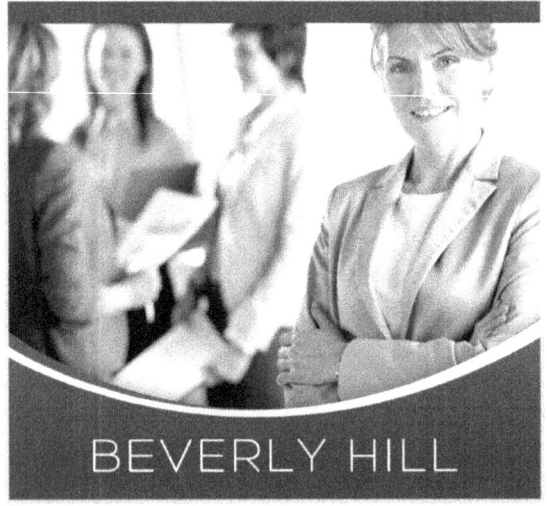

Go to amazon.com to check out the rest of 'MIDDLE AGE CAREER CHANGE: HOW TO TURN YOUR LIFE PASSION INTO A CAREER'

Check Out My Other Books

Below you'll find some of my other popular books that are popular on Amazon and Kindle as well. Simply go to amazon.com to check out the books below. Alternatively, you can visit my author page on Amazon to see other work done by me.

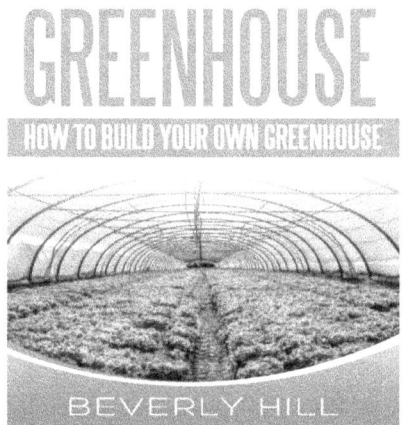

GREENHOUSE: HOW TO BUILD YOUR OWN GREENHOUSE.

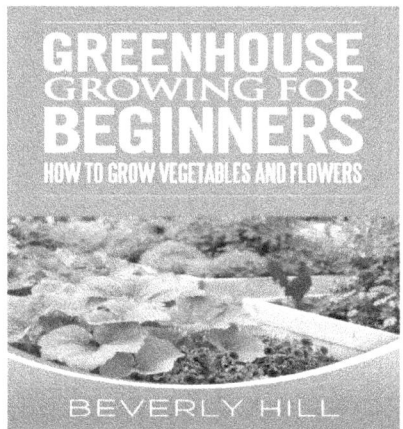

GREENHOUSE GROWING FOR BEGINNERS; HOW TO GROW VEGETABLES AND FLOWERS.

BONUS: SUBSCRIBE TO THE FREE BOOK

Beginners Guide to Yoga & Meditation

"Stressed out? Do You Feel Like The World Is Crashing Down Around You? Want To Take A Vacation That Will Relax Your Mind, Body And Spirit? Well this Easy To Read Step By Step

E-Book Makes It All Possible!"

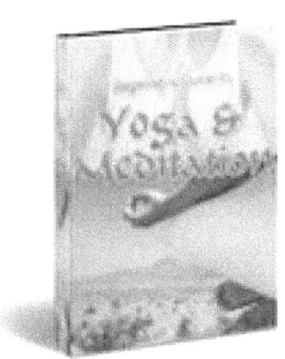

Instructions on how to join our mailing list, and receive a free copy of "Yoga and Meditation" can be found in any of my Kindle eBooks.

NOTES

NOTES

NOTES

NOTES

NOTES

NOTES

www.ingramcontent.com/pod-product-compliance
Lightning Source LLC
Chambersburg PA
CBHW071549170526
45166CB00004B/1604